THE NATURE DOCTOR

A MANUAL OF TRADITIONAL AND COMPLEMENTARY MEDICINE